MOLASES BLACKSTRAP

HEALTH BENEFITS AND NUTRITIONAL FACTS

TERRANCE B. WITNEY

Table of Contents

CHAPTER ONE

What is Molasses?

Molasses is a thick, dim, and gooey syrup that is a result of the sugar refining process. It is regularly delivered from sugarcane or sugar beet during the extraction of sugar. The interaction includes reducing the sugarcane or sugar beet juice to separate the sugar gems. As the juice is heated up, the sugar takes shape and is eliminated from the fluid. The excess fluid, which is plentiful in nutrients, minerals, and different mixtures, becomes molasses.

Molasses comes in various assortments in view of how frequently the sugar has been extricated from the first squeeze. The various sorts of molasses include:

* Light Molasses: This is the main molasses delivered during the sugar extraction process. It has a lighter tone and a better, milder flavor. It's generally expected utilized in baking and cooking.

* Dull Molasses: Dim molasses is the consequence of a second round of bubbling after light molasses has been taken out. It has a more strong flavor and hazier variety because of the expanded caramelization of sugars.

* Blackstrap Molasses: This is the thickest and most obscure kind of molasses. It's the after effect of the third and last bubbling of the sugar remove. Blackstrap molasses has the most extraordinary flavor and is plentiful in minerals like iron, calcium, and potassium. It's

not unexpected utilized as a nourishing enhancement.

Authentic Foundation of molasses

The historical backdrop of molasses is entwined with the historical backdrop of sugar creation, exchange, and imperialism. Here is a concise outline of the verifiable foundation of molasses:

Antiquated Times: The extraction of sugar from sugarcane is accepted to have begun in old India, where sugarcane was first developed. The information on sugar creation spread to different districts, including the Center East and Mediterranean, through shipping lanes.

Middle age and Renaissance Europe: Sugar turned into a profoundly sought-after product in middle age Europe, however it was at first an extravagance thing because of its unique case and the perplexing system of refining it. As shipping lanes extended, sugar creation expanded, and procedures for refining sugar gotten to the next level.

Pilgrim Time and the Caribbean: In the fifteenth and sixteenth hundreds of years, European provincial powers, especially the Portuguese, Spanish, Dutch, French, and English, laid out sugarcane manors in the Caribbean and the Americas. These manors required serious work, which prompted the overseas slave exchange as oppressed Africans were brought to deal with these estates. The creation of sugar yielded molasses as a side-effect.

Three-sided Exchange: The sugar estates in the Caribbean and the Americas were important for the more extensive three-sided exchange framework. Molasses assumed a part in this exchange too. Molasses was transported to New Britain, where it was utilized in the creation of rum. This rum was then exchanged for subjugated Africans in West Africa, shaping one leg of the three-sided shipping lane.

American Transformation: Molasses likewise assumed a part in the American Upset. The English forced charges on molasses and different products through acts,.

Post-Unrest and Industrialization: After the American Upheaval, the creation and utilization of molasses kept on extending. It was utilized as a sugar, in cooking, and as a vital fixing in rum creation. The development of industrialization and progressions in sugar refining innovation further expanded the accessibility of molasses.

Current Purposes: Over the long haul, the job of molasses in modern cycles moved, and its utilization in food items turned out to be more normal. Molasses is utilized in different culinary applications, from baking and cooking to the development of sauces, marinades, and, surprisingly, specific sorts of animals feed.

CHAPTER TWO

Significance and Utilizations

Molasses has an assortment of significance and utilizations, both by and large and in current times. Here are a portion of the critical parts of its significance and utilizations:

Culinary Purposes

Baking: Molasses is a typical fixing in baking, particularly in recipes like gingerbread, molasses treats, and dull breads. It adds a particular flavor and wetness to heated merchandise.

Sauces and Marinades: Molasses is utilized in the planning of sauces, marinades, and coatings for dishes like grill ribs, barbecued meats, and cooked vegetables. Its profound, rich flavor supplements exquisite dishes.

Improving Specialist

Normal Sugar: Molasses can be utilized as a characteristic sugar in different dishes and drinks. While it tastes areas of strength for really, confers a remarkable pleasantness that can be engaging in specific settings.

Nourishing Enhancement

Blackstrap Molasses: Blackstrap molasses, the most focused kind of molasses, is much of the time considered a wholesome enhancement because of its high mineral substance. It contains critical measures of iron, calcium, magnesium, and potassium. Certain individuals integrate blackstrap molasses into their weight control plans to assist with meeting their dietary requirements.

Rum Creation

Refining: Molasses is a vital fixing in the development of rum. Matured molasses is refined to make rum, a famous cocktail. Various kinds of molasses can add to varieties in the flavor and attributes of the last rum item.

Domesticated animals Feed

Creature Feed: Molasses is in some cases utilized as a fixing in animals feed, especially for creatures like cows and ponies. It can improve the taste and agreeability of feed, making it more interesting to creatures.

Wellbeing and Health

Iron Source: Blackstrap molasses is in many cases advanced as a characteristic wellspring of iron, making it possibly gainful for people with lack of iron pallor.

Mineral Enhancement

notwithstanding iron, blackstrap molasses contains different minerals that can add to by and large wholesome admission.

Home Cures

People Medication: Molasses has been utilized in customary society solutions for different purposes, like mitigating sore throats or easing obstruction.

Modern Applications

Modern Cycles: Molasses is utilized in modern cycles past food and drink creation. It has been used in the development of specific synthetic compounds, drugs, and, surprisingly, as a part in some animals takes care of.

Authentic Importance:

Provincial Exchange: Molasses assumed a huge part in verifiable exchange designs, including the three-sided exchange between Europe, Africa, and the Americas. It was a critical part in the creation of rum, which had financial ramifications for provincial abilities.

CHAPTER THREE

Kinds of Molasses

There are a few kinds of molasses, each delivered at various phases of the sugar extraction process. The sorts of molasses are classified in light of their variety, flavor, and dietary substance. Here are the primary sorts of molasses:

* Light Molasses:

Otherwise called "Barbados" or "first" molasses.

This is the primary molasses created during the sugar extraction process.

It has a lighter tone and a milder, better flavor contrasted with different kinds.

Utilized in baking, marinades, and as an overall sugar.

* Dim Molasses:

Made after the main round of sugar extraction.

Dull molasses has a more grounded, more vigorous flavor and a hazier variety because of additional caramelization of sugars.

Utilized in gingerbread, heated beans, and as a flavor enhancer in different dishes.

* Blackstrap Molasses:

Created after the third and last round of sugar extraction.

The most obscure and thickest kind of molasses.

Blackstrap molasses has the most extraordinary flavor and is extremely supplement thick, containing higher measures of minerals like iron, calcium, and magnesium.

Frequently utilized as a wholesome enhancement and added to recipes for its medical advantages.

* Sulfured Molasses:

Molasses that has been treated with sulfur dioxide as an additive.

The sulfur dioxide keeps up with the molasses' tone and expands its timeframe of realistic usability.

Sulfured molasses might have a somewhat unique flavor contrasted with unsulfured molasses.

* Unsulfured Molasses:

Molasses that has not been treated with sulfur dioxide.

Thought about a more regular and unadulterated type of molasses.

Frequently liked for its cleaner taste and potential medical advantages.

Stick Molasses:

Gotten from sugarcane juice during the sugar extraction process.

The most widely recognized kind of molasses that anyone could hope to find.

Assortments like light, dull, and blackstrap stick molasses are delivered.

* Beet Molasses:

Produced using sugar beet handling, like sugarcane molasses.

By and large lighter in variety and milder in flavor than stick molasses.

Utilized in food creation and animals feed.

Extravagant Molasses:

An excellent molasses that falls among light and dull molasses concerning variety and flavor.

Frequently utilized in baking and cooking where a more adjusted flavor is wanted

* Creation Cycle

The creation interaction of molasses is firmly connected to the extraction of sugar from sugarcane or sugar beet. Here is an outline of the creation cycle of molasses:

Collecting and Arrangement

Sugarcane or sugar beet plants are collected when they have arrived at development. Sugarcane is commonly reaped by slicing the stalks near the ground, while sugar beets are removed.

The reaped plants are shipped to the handling office for additional arrangement.

* Extraction of Sugar Juice:

The gathered sugarcane or sugar beet plants are cleaned, washed, and squashed to extricate their juices. This juice contains water, sugars, and other dissolvable parts.

* Explanation:

The separated juice is then explained to eliminate pollutions like soil, garbage, and other non-sugar parts. This can include processes like filtration and settling.

Bubbling and Vanishing:

The explained juice is then warmed and bubbled to focus the sugar content. As the juice bubbles, water dissipates, and the sugars become more focused.

* Sugar Crystallization:

During the bubbling system, sugar precious stones start to shape as the sugar focus increments. These precious stones are isolated from the fluid through processes like centrifugation or filtration.

* First Molasses Creation:

After the underlying round of sugar crystallization, the leftover fluid is called first molasses. This molasses is lighter in variety and better in taste because of the lower centralization of sugar.

Second Bubbling and Sugar Extraction: The fluid that remaining parts after the principal round of sugar crystallization is bubbled again to separate more sugar precious stones. This cycle yields more obscure molasses with a more grounded flavor.

* Second Molasses Creation:

The fluid coming about because of the subsequent bubbling is known as second molasses or dim molasses. It's utilized in different culinary applications and has a more hearty flavor.

* Third Bubbling and Sugar Extraction:

Now and again, the leftover fluid is bubbled again to extricate any excess sugar. This interaction yields the haziest and thickest molasses, known as blackstrap molasses.

CHAPTER FOUR

Blackstrap Molasses Creation

The fluid got from the third bubbling is blackstrap molasses. It has the most minimal sugar content yet is plentiful in minerals and supplements.

* Cooling and Bundling:

After the fitting molasses type has been created, the fluid is cooled and bundled for conveyance. It very well may be sold in compartments going from containers to bigger mass holders.

Nourishing Substance

The nourishing substance of molasses changes in view of the sort of molasses and its creation cycle. By and large, molasses is a wellspring of carbs, especially sugars, yet it likewise contains a few minerals and nutrients. Here is an outline of the dietary substance of an ordinary serving (1 tablespoon) of blackstrap molasses:

Calories: Around 47 calories

Sugars: Around 12 grams

Sugars: Around 9.5 grams (essentially sucrose)

Dietary Fiber: Unimportant sum

Minerals:

Iron: Around 3.5 mg (around 19% of the suggested day to day admission for grown-ups)

Calcium: Around 172 mg (around 17% of the suggested everyday admission for grown-ups)

Magnesium: Around 48 mg (around 12% of the suggested day

to day consumption for grown-ups)

Potassium: Around 293 mg

Manganese: Around 0.8 mg (around 34% of the suggested day to day consumption for grown-ups)

Nutrients:

Vitamin B6 (Pyridoxine): Around 0.09 mg (around 7% of the suggested everyday admission for grown-ups)

Niacin (Vitamin B3): Roughly 0.45 mg (around 3% of the suggested day to day admission for grown-ups)

Pantothenic Corrosive (Vitamin B5): Around 0.26 mg (around 5% of the suggested everyday admission for grown-ups)

It's essential to take note of that the dietary benefits can differ marginally founded on the particular brand and handling of the molasses. Blackstrap molasses is especially supplement thick contrasted with different sorts of molasses because of its numerous rounds of sugar extraction and the grouping of minerals during the bubbling system.

While integrating molasses into your eating regimen, particularly blackstrap molasses, it can give huge measures of specific minerals like iron, calcium, and magnesium, which can be valuable for those with supplement inadequacies. Be that as it may, molasses is likewise generally high in sugar and calories, so it ought to be consumed with some restraint, particularly assuming you're aware of your sugar consumption or have dietary limitations

Sauces and Marinades:

Molasses is a critical fixing in grill sauces, contributing a sweet, smoky flavor and a rich tone to the sauce.

It can likewise be utilized to make marinades for meats, giving both flavor and a somewhat caramelized outside when cooked.

Prepared Beans:

Molasses is a conventional part of heated beans, adding a sweet and flavorful component to the dish.

Its rich flavor supplements the generous kinds of beans and different fixings.

Coatings and Fixings:

Molasses-based coatings can be brushed onto broiled meats, like ham or chicken, for a delightful caramelized finish.

Showering molasses over flapjacks, waffles, or cereal can give a characteristic and one of a kind pleasantness.

Confections and Desserts:

Molasses is utilized in the creation of different confections, like taffy and fudges, adding to their flavor and surface.

Smoothies and Refreshments:

A modest quantity of molasses can be added to smoothies for a smidgen of pleasantness and an interesting flavor profile.

It can likewise be utilized as a characteristic sugar in hot refreshments like tea or espresso.

Salad Dressings:

Molasses can be integrated into vinaigrettes or dressings, offsetting the sharpness with its sweet and hearty notes.

Grains and Cereals:

Blending molasses into oats, porridge, or yogurt can give a delightful contort to breakfast dishes.

Veggie lover and Vegetarian Dishes:

Molasses can be utilized to add profundity of flavor to veggie lover and vegetarian dishes, like stews, soups, and cooked vegetables.

Pastries:

Molasses can be utilized as a fixing in pastries like pies, puddings, and frozen yogurts, offering a particular taste and a more obscure tint

CHAPTER FIVE

Modern Applications

Notwithstanding its culinary purposes, molasses has different modern applications in various areas. A portion of these applications exploit its compound properties, supplement content, and thickness. The following are a couple of instances of how molasses is utilized in different modern settings:

Animals Feed and Creature Nourishment:

Molasses is much of the time remembered for domesticated animals feed to further develop acceptability and increment energy content.

It very well may be added to creature takes care of, especially for cows, as a wellspring of sugars and energy.

Maturation and Liquor Creation:

Molasses is a critical fixing in the development of cocktails like rum.

Yeast is added to molasses to go through maturation, prompting the development of ethanol and different results.

Microbial Development:

In microbial science and biotechnology, molasses can act as a development mechanism for the development of different microorganisms.

Its starch content gives a supplement source to organisms utilized in processes like biofuel creation, compound combination, and other modern applications.

Modern Maturation Cycles:

Molasses can be utilized as a substrate for modern maturation processes, where microorganisms convert sugars into valuable items like compounds, natural acids, and biofuels.

Bioremediation:

Molasses has been utilized in bioremediation cycles to animate the development of microorganisms that assist with separating and remediate pollutants in soil and water.

De-icing Arrangements:

Because of its consistency and hygroscopic properties (capacity to assimilate dampness), molasses can be utilized in de-icing answers for work on their viability in forestalling ice arrangement on streets and walkways.

Firefighting Froth:

At times, molasses has been integrated into firefighting froth definitions to upgrade their viability in stifling flames.

Development Industry:

Molasses-based arrangements have been utilized as a part in dust suppressants utilized in development and mining exercises.

Substance Creation:

Molasses can act as a feedstock in the development of specific synthetic substances, like lactic corrosive and citrus extract.

Fake Trap and Draws:

Molasses is once in a while utilized in the creation of fishing trap and draws, as its fragrance can draw in fish

Molasses in Medication

Molasses has been generally utilized in customary medication and is frequently considered for its potential medical advantages because of its supplement content.

Nonetheless, it's essential to take note of that logical examination on the restorative purposes of molasses is restricted, and any potential advantages ought to be drawn nearer with alert. Here are a few manners by which molasses has been related with restorative or wellbeing related utilizes:

Iron Hotspot for Sickliness:

Blackstrap molasses is many times advanced as a characteristic wellspring of iron and different minerals, making it possibly helpful for people with lack of iron paleness.

Iron is a crucial part of hemoglobin, which conveys oxygen in the blood. Paleness happens when there's a lack of iron, prompting weakness and different side effects.

Wholesome Supplementation:

Blackstrap molasses is plentiful in minerals like calcium, magnesium, and potassium, which are fundamental for different physical processes.

Certain individuals use blackstrap molasses as a dietary enhancement to assist with meeting their healthful requirements, especially for minerals that might be deficient in their weight control plans.

Stomach related Wellbeing:

In customary medication, molasses has been utilized as a solution for stomach related issues, like clogging.

The fiber content in molasses might make a gentle diuretic

difference, helping with standard solid discharges.

Mitigating Properties:

A few defenders recommend that the cell reinforcements and minerals present in molasses, like magnesium and manganese, may add to its possible calming impacts.

Bone Wellbeing:

Calcium and magnesium, both tracked down in molasses, are significant for keeping up areas of strength for with.

A few people use molasses as a wellspring of these minerals to help bone wellbeing.

It's essential to move toward the utilization of molasses for restorative purposes with alert and counsel a medical services proficient prior to making any huge dietary changes or involving it as an enhancement. While molasses contains specific supplements that can add to generally wellbeing, it ought not be utilized as a substitute for clinical treatment or recommended meds

Social and Culinary

Molasses plays played critical parts in different societies and cooking styles all over the planet. Its unmistakable flavor and flexibility have made it a staple fixing in customary dishes and culinary practices. This is a gander at the way molasses is utilized socially and in culinary settings

CHAPTER SIX

Social Importance

* North American Food:

In the US and Canada, molasses has verifiable and social importance. Molasses was a critical fixing in pioneer American baking, utilized in recipes like gingerbread and heated beans.

Molasses is related with conventional Southern food, especially in dishes like molasses treats, cornbread, and bar-b-que sauces.

* Caribbean Cooking:

In Caribbean cooking, molasses is frequently used to make tasty marinades, coatings, and sauces for meats and fish.

It's likewise a vital fixing in the creation of rum, which has profound social connections to the locale.

* Center Eastern and Mediterranean Cooking:

Molasses, known as "dibs" in Arabic, is a typical fixing in Center Eastern and Mediterranean cooking.

It's utilized to improve dishes like cakes, treats, and refreshments. One model is "dibs el kharroub" or carob molasses, which is famous in the district.

* Indian Cooking:

Molasses is utilized in Latin American foods to add profundity of flavor to dishes like sauces, stews, and certain desserts.

In Brazil, molasses called "rapadura" is utilized to make conventional confections and desserts.

* Sauces and Marinades:

Molasses-based sauces are utilized in barbecuing and grilling to add a sweet and tart flavor to meats.

Likewise utilized as a base for marinades upgrade the flavor and surface of barbecued or cooked dishes.

* Sweets:

Molasses is integrated into various treats, including pies, puddings, cakes, and frozen yogurts.

Its extraordinary flavor can make complex taste profiles in sweet treats.

* Coatings and Garnishes:

Molasses-based coats are brushed onto simmered meats, making a caramelized hull and rich tone.

Sprinkling molasses over breakfast dishes, flapjacks, or waffles can add a novel touch.

* Customary Dishes:

Molasses is a fundamental fixing in famous dishes like Boston heated beans, a generous and delightful dish made with naval force beans and molasses.

In certain societies, molasses is utilized to make taffy or confections, displaying its adaptability.

* Refreshments:

Molasses is some of the time utilized as a sugar or enhancing specialist in hot drinks like tea or espresso.

It tends to be integrated into mixed drinks and blended beverages to add profundity and intricacy.

The utilization of molasses in various societies and culinary practices features its flexibility and capacity to add to many dishes. Whether it's adding a dash of pleasantness or a profundity of flavor, molasses stays a significant fixing in kitchens all over the planet.

Ecological Effect

The ecological effect of molasses creation and utilization can shift contingent upon elements like the wellspring of the molasses (sugarcane or sugar beet), creation techniques, transportation, and waste administration. Here are a few viewpoints to consider with respect to the ecological effect of molasses:

Horticultural Practices:

The development of sugarcane and sugar beets requires land, water, and energy assets. Horticulture can add to deforestation, living space annihilation, and water shortage in specific locales.

The utilization of pesticides, herbicides, and composts in ordinary cultivating practices might possibly prompt ecological contamination and soil debasement.

Water Use:

Sugarcane and sugar beet development require huge measures of water, which can strain neighborhood water assets, particularly in locales with water shortage issues.

Energy Power:

The handling of sugarcane or sugar beet into molasses includes energy-serious cycles like pounding, bubbling, and vanishing. The energy sources utilized for these cycles can influence fossil fuel byproducts.

Waste and Results:

Molasses creation is a result of the sugar extraction process. While this diminishes squander, there are still side-effects from the handling of sugarcane or sugar beets that should be made due, like bagasse (sugarcane fiber) and beet mash.

Transportation:

The transportation of sugarcane, sugar beets, and molasses includes energy utilization and can add to ozone depleting substance discharges on the off chance that not oversaw productively.

Biodiversity and Environments:

Agrarian extension, especially for sugarcane, can prompt deforestation and natural surroundings misfortune, influencing biodiversity and environments.

Carbon Impression:

The carbon impression of molasses creation incorporates

discharges from horticulture, handling, transportation, and energy use. Feasible practices, like decreasing energy utilization and using environmentally friendly power sources, can moderate these discharges.

Feasible Practices:

A few sugar and molasses makers are taking on reasonable practices to limit their natural effect. This incorporates utilizing natural cultivating techniques, improving water use, and carrying out squander the executives procedures.

Food Framework Effect:

The utilization of molasses, particularly in huge amounts, can add to the in general ecological effect of the food framework.

Offsetting abstains from food considering supportability is significant.

Bundling and Circulation:

The bundling and circulation of molasses can produce squander, particularly if non-recyclable materials are utilized. Selecting manageable bundling choices can assist with diminishing ecological effect

CHAPTER SEVEN

Molasses and Soil Wellbeing

Molasses can emphatically affect soil wellbeing when utilized appropriately as a feature of an exhaustive soil the executives methodology. It is many times utilized as a change or added substance to further develop soil structure, microbial movement, and supplement accessibility. Here are a few manners by which molasses can add to soil wellbeing:

Microbial Movement: Molasses is a wellspring of straightforward sugars, which can act as a food hotspot for useful soil microorganisms, including microscopic organisms and parasites. Adding molasses to the dirt can invigorate microbial development and action, prompting worked on supplement cycling and natural matter disintegration.

Organic Variety: Improving microbial action in the dirt through molasses application can build the variety of soil microorganisms. A different microbial local area can add to supplement accessibility, illness concealment, and generally speaking soil environment wellbeing.

Supplement Delivery: The microbial breakdown of molasses and natural matter can deliver supplements in a structure that plants can promptly retain. This can work on supplement accessibility and diminish the requirement for engineered composts.

Soil Construction: Molasses can assist with further developing soil structure by advancing the accumulation of soil particles. This prompts better water penetration, seepage, and air circulation, which are urgent for root advancement and plant development.

pH Guideline: Molasses has a somewhat acidic pH, and its application can assist with adjusting soil pH levels in basic soils. Legitimate pH levels are significant for supplement accessibility and the development of soil creatures.

Manure Enactment: When added to compost heaps, molasses can speed up the decay interaction by giving a promptly accessible carbon hotspot for microorganisms. This can bring about quicker fertilizing the soil and the creation of supplement rich manure.

Rhizosphere Improvement: Molasses can advance the improvement of the rhizosphere, the region encompassing plant roots where a perplexing cooperation between plants, soil, and microorganisms happens. This can prompt better supplement take-up and establish wellbeing.

THE END